10 mindful minutes

a journal

also by goldie hawn

A LOTUS GROWS IN THE MUD: A MEMOIR

with Wendy Holden

10 MINDFUL MINUTES

with Wendy Holden

10 mindful minutes
a journal

Goldie Hawn
with Jennifer Repo

A PERIGEE BOOK

A PERIGEE BOOK
Published by the Penguin Group
Penguin Group (USA) LLC
375 Hudson Street, New York, New York 10014

USA · Canada · UK · Ireland · Australia · New Zealand · India · South Africa · China

penguin.com

A Penguin Random House Company

10 MINDFUL MINUTES: A JOURNAL

ISBN: 978-0-399-17491-9

This book has been registered with the Library of Congress.

First edition: June 2015

PRINTED IN THE UNITED STATES OF AMERICA

10   9   8   7   6   5   4   3   2   1

Text design by Tiffany Estreicher
Illustrations by Durell Godfrey

To those who walk the path of self-discovery, challenging the status quo for a happier life.

And to my grandchildren, with the hope that we can leave them a more peaceful, mindful world.

contents

Discovering Empathy

Becoming Compassionate

Tending to Kindness

what we think is
what we create

*There are no mistakes. The events we bring upon ourselves,
no matter how unpleasant, are necessary in order to learn what
we need to learn; whatever steps we take, they're necessary to
reach the places we've chosen to go.*

—Richard Bach

It was an unusually rainy day in Los Angeles. I welcomed the indoor
time, when I could cozy up under a blanket and read whatever I
liked. At one point, my eyes drifted off the page to watch the rain
against the window. It was then I noticed my volumes of diaries,
lined up on the bookshelf. It was the perfect day to indulge my curiosity and so I started to read from the first book, dated 1970. I wanted
to see what the younger Goldie wrote about and what I was doing,
thinking, and feeling at that time.

Without really realizing it, I found myself looking for insights to
who I was—or at least who I thought I was—back then. Sometimes
funny, mostly somber, but always illuminating, these pages reminded

me of my struggles and disappointments. (Why is it that in our youth we write so often about bad, sad times and not so much about the happy ones?) Some of the pages were literally tearstained. It was almost like reading about some other young person's laments on love, loss, self-worth, and fear. It was evident that I was trying to make sense of these emotions and to understand more about myself. It certainly appeared that I'd been on an emotional roller coaster, with the ups and downs of my personal and professional lives raw on the page.

I skipped forward a few decades to find that my more recent reflections were quite different. A little more mature, perhaps, but clearly reflecting the effort I made to determine my true objectives— to be happy and well—through self-discovery and deepening my spiritual life. In these later diaries I seldom wrote about my sorry state, but had come to recognize my connection to a greater consciousness. I was tuning in to the wonder and the preciousness of life, with gratitude. I was clearly feeling more connected, more present, and much happier.

This change of spirit didn't happen on its own. Reading these journals just confirmed what I already know, but sometimes forget— that it took intention on my part to learn to deal with my fears, realize my potential, become attuned to others, and understand the liberation of forgiveness.

I believe that what we think is what we create. With committed intention you can replace negative self-talk with positive affirmation. As you commit to your own journal, you will come to understand that awareness of your destructive thoughts or tendencies is the first step toward change. Your own words can become a means to discover and open up the channels to your greatest potential.

I also think that this journal can be an important step to becoming more mindful. As you reflect on the lessons and respond to the questions here, your mind will be opened to new perspectives and, just as it did for me, journaling fearlessly will give you a deeper understanding of yourself. I guarantee that you will relish the experience.

Since it can be intimidating to face a blank page, this guided journal offers prompts, questions, and simple meditations to get you started.

Before you begin to write, sit quietly by yourself. Close your eyes and simply focus on your breathing. Quiet your mind as best you can. Although your mind will at first be overwhelmed with its own busyness, allow those thoughts to become clouds and let them drift away. Return to your breath until you feel calm and relaxed. This is the point when you are most in tune with yourself.

Write slowly and with as much clarity as you can. Keep it simple. No one is judging your journal on its literary merit. And you don't want to be judging yourself. When you write deliberately and mindfully you will be less frenzied and more focused. If you feel blocked, don't be hard on yourself. There are no deadlines. Take a break and come back with a fresh perspective and be more open to the process. (Even while writing this introduction, I had to take some time to let my mind drift, to think about other things, have some lunch, and then pick up my pen again.)

Good luck, have fun, and remember to try not to edit yourself. These are your pages, and you have nothing to hide, especially from yourself.

In grammar school I often signed my homework assignments, "With love, Goldie." When my mother asked me why, I answered, "Because I love my teacher."

I think it only fitting to sign off with the same sentiment to you.

With love, Goldie

cultivating
optimism

Optimism has emotional benefits far beyond giving us more happiness in the moment and more hope for a positive future; it also helps relationships survive.

—10 Mindful Minutes

I am still determined to be cheerful and to be happy in whatever situation I may be, for I have also learnt from experience that the greater part of our happiness or misery depends upon our dispositions, and not upon our circumstances.

—Martha Washington

How we talk to ourselves deeply affects how we see the world. We can actually begin to change the pathways in the brain with a short mindful exercise I call "Creating Attitude."

1. Sit comfortably either in a chair or on a cushion. Make sure you're sitting nice and tall.

2. Place your palms facedown on top of your thighs.

3. Close your eyes and take a deep inhale; and as you exhale, imagine emptying your mind of all its thoughts. It is the nature of the mind to think, so these thoughts will come. Simply let them pass as though they're floating down a river. Try not to judge yourself or self-criticize. Or get caught up in your unresolved problems of the day.

4. Focus on your breath, your inhales and exhales. This relaxes both the mind and the body. Do this a few times.

5. Here are a few suggested phrases to start saying to yourself. You can create your own or use these.

I love my life.

I have everything I need right now.

Everything is exactly as it should be right now.

Today is a great day.

I think positively in difficult or stressful situations.

I look for the good in everything that happens.

power of possibility

*From the age of eleven, whenever someone asked me what
I wanted to be when I grew up, I'd say simply, "Happy."*
—*10 Mindful Minutes*

Close your eyes. Take a deep breath and as you exhale, think about emptying the mind of all thoughts. Imagine that your mind is like a vase full of water. With each exhale imagine the water slowly draining out of the vase. With your eyes still closed, think back to when you were a child, when life was carefree and you had no responsibilities and the possibilities were endless. What brought you joy? What were your hopes and dreams? What was your favorite thing to do? What did you most want to do? Open your eyes and, without hesitation, start writing about what you wanted for yourself, what you wanted to do or be.

Now look back and read what you wrote. Remember that is still you. You have the power to create what you want. As you go through your day, try to remember that feeling of childhood optimism—when the whole world was wide open to you! It still is!

a mindful do-over

*Optimism acts like a resiliency vaccine that enables us to bounce
back from emotional and physical difficulties more easily.*
—*10 Mindful Minutes*

We all have moments throughout the day when something doesn't
go our way. Think about a situation recently that didn't go your way.
How did you react? Be honest. How did you feel about how you
handled it? If you had a do-over, how could you have been more
mindful of your words or actions?

half full or half empty?

*Sometimes the choices we make are good, and sometimes
they are bad. Sometimes the fear of making a bad choice
prevents us from making any choice at all.*

—A Lotus Grows in the Mud

Things don't always go the way we want—or think we want. Consider what positive results might come out of *not* getting what you want. This is an opportunity to see the glass as *half full* or *half empty*. What's your perspective?

I wanted

....

....

....

....

....

What I got was

....

....

....

....

....

I wanted

....

....

....

....

....

What I got was

....

....

....

....

....

saying yes

*Positive emotions have the added bonus of allowing
us to take in more information and therefore see a wider
range of solutions to problems.*
—*10 Mindful Minutes*

Your spouse asked for a date night and you declined. Or your children wanted you to read to them but you complained that you were too tired.

How many times do you say the word "no" throughout your day? Maybe you say it often to your children, your spouse, or your friends when they ask you to do something.

Recall one of the times you said no. Just observe this and try not to edit or criticize yourself.

What could have happened if you had said yes?

Write down something positive that would have come out of it. How could your "yes" have made you feel happier?

any day happiness

It's a matter of holding positive attitudes, which include
seeing a negative situation as an opportunity for growth, focusing
on a brighter future, practicing gratitude, and laughing as
much as possible whenever possible.

—10 Mindful Minutes

In *10 Mindful Minutes*, I describe an activity called "Rainy Day Blues,"
in which you and your children pretend it's raining outside. I suggest
acting out positive responses such as jumping up and down in a
puddle or throwing back your head to feel the rain on your face. Now
here is an activity just for you.

Whatever the weather, take just a few minutes for yourself and go
outside. Focus on simple things like the air on your skin, the leaves
on the trees, the sweet smell of the air as you take a long, deep breath
in and slowly exhale.

Now write about how you are *feeling.*

train your brain

*Creating more positive than negative thoughts
fosters greater optimism, which allows us to see a light at
the end of our particular tunnel.*
—10 Mindful Minutes

You can train your brain. Even as you think of negative things in your life you can turn them around to find the positive aspects. Your brain will like this and you will generate more happiness pathways. Write down some of your negative experiences, and then find a way to give them a more positive outcome. For instance, you could focus on problems at work or home, or even on your internal negative-speak, such as "I am not good enough" or "I can't do this very well."

Your negative experience

....

....

....

Find the positive in this experience

....

....

....

....

....

Your negative experience

....

....

....

....

....

Find the positive in this experience

....

....

....

....

....

savoring
happiness

*If we are happy, relaxed, and curious . . .
our brains open like a flower.*

—*10 Mindful Minutes*

Learn to enjoy every minute of your life.
Be happy now. Don't wait for something outside of
yourself to make you happy in the future. Think
how really precious is the time you have to spend,
whether it's at work or with your family. Every
minute should be enjoyed and savored.

—Earl Nightingale

1. Sit comfortably either in a chair or on a cushion. Make sure you're sitting nice and tall.

2. Place your palms facedown on top of your thighs.

3. Close your eyes and focus on your breath, your inhales and exhales. When you inhale, bring in the positive. When you exhale, let go of the negative. Do this a few times until you feel relaxed.

4. Think about something that went well for you recently, even a simple experience like eating a sweet, juicy peach. Spend time recalling this experience. Enjoy the unhurried appreciation of joy. Savor it.

happy thoughts

*Savoring is vital to love, friendship, physical and
mental health, creativity, and spirituality. Put simply, it
expands our heart's capacity for joy.*
—10 *Mindful Minutes*

Recall some of the happiest times in your life. Maybe it was the birth
of a child, your wedding day, or when you received a well-deserved
job promotion. Write about how you really felt on two of these occa-
sions. Do you remember the unending joy coursing through your
body? Did you feel elated? Did you feel connected to something
bigger than yourself?

I felt happy when

....

....

....

....

I felt happy when

....

....

....

....

While these memories are still fresh in your mind, write about what makes you happy at this time in your life. This exercise will make you more mindful of the wellspring of happiness from which you can draw at any time.

I am happy when

....

....

....

....

I am happy when

....

....

....

....

rediscovering you!

The key is to look at our gifts, understand their
power, and modulate them realistically. Understand
how important it is to honor them.

—A Lotus Grows in the Mud

Write about a time when you felt attractive, vibrant, and free. Where were you?

As time goes on we sometimes lose our sense of vitality because of the burdens of everyday living. Sit quietly and focus on a time when you felt attractive, vibrant, and free. You will enliven your spirit as you recall these precious moments—and rediscover the real you.

happiness is within

*If someone asks me what makes me happiest, it is never anything
I can quantify like a house or a possession or something I can
touch. It is the spirit of the human being, which can fill me with
more joy than anything in the world.*

—*A Lotus Grows in the Mud*

In *10 Mindful Minutes*, I write about the phenomenon called "hedonistic treadmill"—the misguided belief that has us thinking that acquiring new toys, gadgets, or whatever will make us happy. Shift your attention to recent experiences that didn't involve material things yet brought you unfettered joy. Note a few of these here:

....

....

....

....

....

creative happiness

Perhaps the most important thing optimism and savoring happiness can do is prevent depression, because they exercise areas of our brains that make us less likely to get depressed, even when facing hard times.

—*10 Mindful Minutes*

Take out an old photograph. It could be a photo from when you were a child or a more recent one of your family. Maybe it's a scenic photograph that simply makes you feel contented. Write about this photo in any way that feels good to you. You might try writing a creative short story or even a fantasy. Or simply recount how you feel when you look at the photograph.

your happy place

I discovered that the landscape of the mind is an endlessly
fascinating place. The more I learned, the more excited I became
about tapping into its almost limitless potential.

—*10 Mindful Minutes*

In *10 Mindful Minutes*, I suggest that you gather items from around
your home and create a "Happiness Box" for you and your children.
It's a wonderful way to create happy memories together. But now I
suggest an activity that is only for you.

Use the spaces in the next few pages to draw or paste images or
write down thoughts and ideas that make you happy. Think of this
space as a mini vision board of all that makes you feel good. You
might cut out an image from a magazine and paste it here—like a
photo of a hot fudge sundae (which is something I would include!),
one of your children's drawings, or a favorite poem or quotation.
Whatever you decide to include, let these pages be an expression of
your "happy place."

attitude of
gratitude

When we focus on how grateful we are for what's right in our lives, even in the midst of challenges, we recognize that a situation isn't totally bleak and give ourselves the energy to move forward.

—*10 Mindful Minutes*

*For me, every hour is grace. And I feel
gratitude in my heart each time I can meet
someone and look at his or her smile.*

—Elie Wiesel

Usually when we sit quietly for these mindfulness moments, we try to empty the mind of all thoughts. But for this one, I want to encourage you to try to recall every single thing you are grateful for.

1. Find a quiet place where you can sit comfortably, undisturbed.

2. Place your palms faceup on top of your thighs. Palms faceup is symbolic of being open to receiving the intention of this mindfulness exercise.

3. Close your eyes and start focusing on your breath. Each inhale and exhale.

4. Begin by thinking about every single thing in your life that you are grateful for.

5. Even if the mind wanders, keep the list going. They might be small things such as being grateful for having more than one pair of shoes. Or being grateful for the smile that someone gave you yesterday.

vitamin g

*I am now convinced that gratitude is a powerful force for our
bodies, minds, and emotions—I call it vitamin G.*

—10 Mindful Minutes

Research has shown that people who feel gratitude tend to be more
content and peaceful. And there is no better way to start your day
than being grateful for what is in your life. For this prompt, I ask you
to write down three things that you are grateful for. Try this for
seven days and then continue if you wish. Notice how your attitude
shifts when you are doing this exercise.

DAY 1

1. ....

2. ....

3. ....

DAY 2

1. ....

2. ....

3. ....

DAY 3

1. ....

2. ....

3. ....

DAY 4

1. ....

2. ....

3. ....

DAY 5

1. ....

2. ....

3. ....

DAY 6

1. ....

2. ....

3. ....

DAY 7

1. ....

2. ....

3. ....

*It is through gratitude for the present moment that
the spiritual dimension of life opens up.*

—Eckhart Tolle

giving back

*I was taught it is our moral duty to give back something
to this world, to say thank you for our gifts.*

—A Lotus Grows in the Mud

Feeling gratitude is wonderful and has many physical, emotional, and spiritual benefits. Expressing gratitude is taking that feeling and sharing it with another human being. In the space provided below, write a letter to someone for whom you feel gratitude. Maybe it's a parent or a mentor or a spiritual adviser. Perhaps it's your child or your child's teacher. Whoever you choose, write this letter from the heart. Then, if you wish, share this letter with the person.

Dear .... :

....

....

....

gratitude symbol

Focusing on what's wrong makes us unhappy and unhealthy, while focusing on what's right boosts body, mind, and spirit. Best of all, gratitude is completely free and takes virtually no time to express.

—10 Mindful Minutes

Find a small object—something small that you can carry with you—a pebble, a token or special coin, a locket picture, or something you create. This can be your gratitude symbol. Throughout the day, when you come across it in your pocket or purse, let it be a reminder to think of one thing to be grateful for. No matter what is going on, take five seconds and feel the gratitude.

*Gratitude makes sense of our past, brings peace
for today, and creates a vision for tomorrow.*

—Melody Beattie

family gratitude

Gratitude is also one of the keys to happy relationships. Through research that spanned two decades, marriage and parenting expert Dr. John Gottman discovered that couples who maintain at least the all-important three-to-one ratio of positive to negative feelings were more likely to have long-lasting relationships.

—10 Mindful Minutes

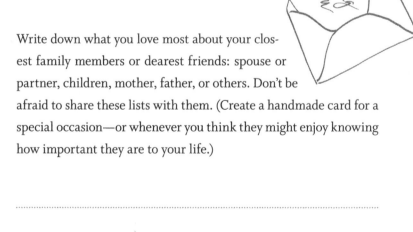

Write down what you love most about your closest family members or dearest friends: spouse or partner, children, mother, father, or others. Don't be afraid to share these lists with them. (Create a handmade card for a special occasion—or whenever you think they might enjoy knowing how important they are to your life.)

thank you

Thank you. *Those two little words convey so much. Thank you means that you've taken the time out to let someone know that you're grateful for something they've said or done.*

—*10 Mindful Minutes*

Psychologists have found that being thankful or appreciative of someone or something is one sure way to increase happiness. Our modern society wants us to think that happiness is found in buying that new television or car—that in purchasing something, we can be happy. However, that kind of happiness—material happiness—is short-lived. The good news is that feeling gratitude is a free and simple way to find inner peace and contentment.

Try this exercise for one day and notice how you feel at the end of the day. Say "thank you" to every single person you encounter today. Look each person in the eye and give a heartfelt show of appreciation. You'll be amazed at how happy this makes the other person feel and how happy you feel as well.

transforming
anger

The true hero is one who conquers his own anger and hatred.

—The Dalai Lama XIV

*Anger is an acid that can do more harm
to the vessel in which it is stored than to
anything on which it is poured.*

—Mark Twain

Mindfulness does not seek to get rid of the feeling of anger, but simply to observe that it is there. To acknowledge that it exists. In the practice below, try to sit with whatever emotions arise, particularly uncomfortable feelings.

1. Sit in a comfortable position, palms facedown.

2. Close your eyes. Begin paying attention to your inhales and exhales.

3. After a few moments of focused breathing, bring to mind something or someone that brings up anger.

4. Recall the situation. Feel the emotions that arise— resentment, jealousy, anger, or fear.

5. Notice if the anger finds a place in your body. Some people feel the anger in their shoulders, some in their hips, and some in their lower back. Simply observe this.

6. Dedicate this meditation as you repeat silently: "May .... be free from pain and sorrow."

feeling it

It is perfectly normal to experience painful feelings,
angry feelings, feelings of resentment. The key, of course,
is how we handle those emotions.

—10 Mindful Minutes

In her book *A Heart as Wide as the World*, Buddhist teacher Sharon Salzberg writes, "When anger is a strong factor of mind, it is often a consequence of projecting outward our inner dissatisfaction." What she is saying is that everything we see around us is in fact a reflection of our emotional state. So for example, even if someone cuts us off in traffic and we feel that person may have wronged us, it is only because we have the perception that all should go smoothly on our ride. The good news is that rather than focus on the person or situation that upset us, we can look inward and ask ourselves, *What are my expectations about this person or situation?*

In the spaces below, complete the sentences as honestly as possible. Write freely and try not to self-edit.

EXAMPLE:

I feel anger when *my husband pays more attention to his phone than to me.*

My expectation is that *I deserve his undivided attention all the time.*

I feel anger when

....

....

My expectation is that

....

....

I feel anger when

....

....

My expectation is that

....

....

something different

*Sometimes, when life gets too hard and crowds in on
you and you become desensitized, you need to remember to just
take time. Go away. Change your surroundings. Put yourself
in a situation where the outcome is uncertain.*

—A Lotus Grows in the Mud

We can't always get away when we'd like. We have families, jobs, and responsibilities. But you can take mini trips that don't require moving from your spot! Try this exercise the next time you get angry. Write a brief statement about what's making you angry—except *write about your anger using your nondominant hand.* You'll be amazed at how the simple act of concentrating on something so different can literally take you away from what you're feeling.

traffic signal

*When we pay attention and remember what is
happening within our brains, we can break the chain of
anger for everyone's well-being.*

—10 Mindful Minutes

In *10 Mindful Minutes*, I suggest playing the "Traffic Signal Game" with children. However, it's also a great one for adults who are wrestling with anger. It's a simple and effective way to calm down.

Imagine a traffic light . . .

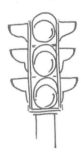

Red: Stop and do mindful breathing.

Yellow: Consider different (and better) ways to respond to a distressing situation.

Green: Try the most mindful response—and see what happens.

Whenever your anger button is pushed, recall the traffic light: pause, breathe, reflect, and *then* act appropriately.

When angry, count ten before you speak;
if very angry, an hundred.

—Thomas Jefferson

what's your trigger?

*Angry outbursts can become habitual; the more you allow
anger to take control, the deeper the brain pathways are carved.
I call them the Grand Canyon of Anger.*

—10 Mindful Minutes

In *10 Mindful Minutes*, I write about the amygdala, the part of the brain that controls the fight-or-flight response. This is what is triggered as a response to anger. Adrenaline is literally flowing through your body and it can become hard to get back to a place of calm. Taking a few moments here, create a list of triggers that you *know* make you angry: when someone cuts you off in traffic or your spouse doesn't put his or her clothes away. Whatever they are, list them. This list might be scarily long—but it's better to get them all down so you can identify them, understand the common factors, and by observing come to conquer your anger.

releasing
sadness

Mindfulness is the conscious awareness of our current thoughts, feelings, and surroundings—and accepting this awareness with openness and curiosity in a nonjudgmental way.

—10 Mindful Minutes

Even a happy life cannot be without a measure of darkness, and the word "happy" would lose its meaning if it were not balanced by sadness. . . . It is therefore far better to take things as they come along, with patience and equanimity.

—Carl Jung

Sadness gives depth. Happiness gives height. Sadness gives roots. Happiness gives branches. Happiness is like a tree going into the sky, and sadness is like the roots going down into the womb of the earth. Both are needed, and the higher a tree goes, the deeper it goes, simultaneously. The bigger the tree, the bigger will be its roots. In fact, it is always in proportion. That's its balance.

—Osho

Experiencing sadness is a part of the human experience. And like most people, we often try to push away or avoid this uncomfortable emotion. The goal of this mindful exercise is to reveal the conditioned response to sadness and observe it for what it is; to try not to change it so that we can have a different relationship with this feeling. Like everything in life, it will pass.

1. Sit comfortably either in a chair or on a cushion. Make sure you're sitting nice and tall.

2. Place your palms faceup on top of your thighs.

3. Close your eyes and take a deep inhale; and as you exhale, observe your thoughts and try to just let them pass

through like clouds in the sky. Sit quietly for a few minutes.

4. Focusing on your breath relaxes both the mind and the body.

5. When you feel ready, bring to mind something that has made you sad. Maybe it's the loss of a loved one or a pet. Maybe it's a conflict with someone you know. Whatever it is, allow the feelings to come. You might cry and that's okay.

6. Visualize healing bright light surrounding the person or situation.

7. With each inhale, breathe in acceptance; with each exhale, breathe out release.

early memories

I have come to learn that going through those periods
of sadness are vitally important to my growth and to my
inner relationship with myself.

—10 Mindful Minutes

What is your earliest memory of feeling sad? Write about what you felt, how you expressed that feeling. Did you cry? Did you share your feelings with anyone?

....

....

....

....

....

....

....

rewriting history

Dark days can follow if we don't become fully aware.
We need to find ways to grow from our down moments instead
of developing a victim mentality.

—*10 Mindful Minutes*

Any feeling of pain, sadness, or anger is uncomfortable. Unfortunately we have become a society that seeks instant remedies to feel better: drugs, alcohol, or unhealthy diversions. But as I've learned, the only way to deal with anger or sadness is to work through it. As well, there comes a point where we must release what we're feeling and let it go. This doesn't mean, however, that we forget a loved one who has died or the loss of something precious to us. On the contrary, the research shows that when people understand their feelings and are able to share them appropriately, they deal with loss better and have healthier relationships.

In just a few lines, write down a situation or event that makes you feel sad.

....

....

....

....

....

....

....

....

Now rewrite this situation in a way that makes you feel less sad.

....

....

....

....

....

....

....

Close your eyes and concentrate on your breath. Visualize the new scene that you've envisioned and with each exhale let go of the sadness.

dance like no one's looking

Dancing gave me something I very much needed as a child. . . . It allowed me to overcome my physical awkwardness as a little girl.

—*A Lotus Grows in the Mud*

I gained confidence as a young girl because dancing gave me a sense of feeling grounded. Maybe you need to have a dance party to feel free. Maybe it will help you feel grounded, too. Forget about everything going on in your life and dance!

When you are home alone, play a song that you love. This will take only a few minutes—or as long as the track of your favorite tune might last! Ignore the thoughts "I shouldn't" or "This is silly" or "I have too much to do." Turn the music up and dance like you've never danced before!

How do you feel now? Write it down.

....

....

your happy playlist

Make a list of all the songs that make you feel happy. Bring them to mind whenever you feel the need. You don't need to download any of these since they are all stored in the "cloud" of your brain, to be retrieved at a moment's notice.

I think I should have no other mortal wants,
if I could always have plenty of music. It seems to
infuse strength into my limbs, and ideas into my
brain. Life seems to go on without effort, when
I am filled with music.

—George Eliot

in your body

I have since come to learn that loss is part of being alive;
it's part of loving. Sadness is just as important as joy. . . . Pain
provides us with the vital ingredient in the genetic makeup of
our character; it is part of the DNA of our philosophy.
—A Lotus Grows in the Mud

Think back to the last time you cried. Maybe you were watching a movie (or even a television show) or reading a book or were responding to a real event or remembrance. Close your eyes and recall the physical sensations that you experienced. Did your throat close up? Did you clench your fists? Did you try to stop yourself from crying?

Write about everything that came to mind: how it felt in your body, how you embraced the feeling or tried to push it away.

sitting with
fear

*Not knowing the outcome of an experience can be
incredibly humbling and refreshingly liberating.*

—A Lotus Grows in the Mud

I have learned over the years that when one's mind is made up, this diminishes fear; knowing what must be done does away with fear.

—Rosa Parks

This powerful visualization technique can be done anywhere and I encourage you to do this whenever you feel the first sign of fear.

1. Sit comfortably either in a chair or on a cushion. Make sure you're sitting nice and tall.

2. Place your palms facedown on top of your thighs.

3. Close your eyes and take a deep inhale; and as you exhale, visualize your thoughts, worries, and anxieties emptying out of the bottom of a pail. The thoughts will still come but try not to get "hooked" on one. Simply observe and let it float away.

4. With each inhale, imagine clear, pure air filling up your body.

5. With each exhale, imagine exhaling the fear in the form of black smoke.

letting go

If we can just let go and trust that things will work out
the way they're supposed to, without trying to control the
outcome, then we can begin to enjoy the moment more fully.
The joy of the freedom it brings becomes more pleasurable
than the experience itself.

—A Lotus Grows in the Mud

Many of our most deep-seated fears stem from childhood experiences or trauma. They are very difficult to face. And much of the time, our fears are driving our daily decisions and can affect our enjoyment of the present moment. In the exercise below, I encourage you to try to name your fears and uncover their origins. From that starting place, you may come to understand that a particular fear might not be related at all to what's going on in your life *right now*, but tied to something that happened to you a long time ago. And with that understanding comes freedom.

List five things you are afraid of:

1. ....

2. ....

3. ....

4. ....

5. ....

For each fear, think back to when you first remember that fearful feeling. If you wrote, "I'm afraid my husband will leave me," this is a fear of rejection or abandonment. When did you first feel rejection? Was it the first time you were dropped off at kindergarten? Was it when your first crush didn't like you back? Write down all the major times in your life when you felt the feelings related to your five fears.

1. ....

2. ....

3. ....

4. ....

5. ....

changing the channel

What you believe isn't important.
What's important is that you believe.
—A Lotus Grows in the Mud

In the previous section you explored the history of your fears and made an honest effort to determine their origins. Now is the time to begin your journal to fearlessness.

One of the best ways to defuse anxiety or fearful thoughts is to block the brain from habituating these feelings. But it's almost impossible to do so without *replacing* those negative ideas with positive thoughts. This action will literally change the pathways in your brain.

Following the example below, write down a fearful thought and immediately replace it with the opposite.

Fearful Thought: I'm afraid my child won't grow up to be successful.

Courageous Thought: My child does well in school and will be happy and successful in life.

FEARFUL THOUGHT:

....

....

....

....

....

....

....

....

....

COURAGEOUS THOUGHT:

....

....

....

....

....

....

....

....

....

walking through fear

Of all the emotions, fear is the one most strongly activated by the amygdala. It is constantly scanning the environment for problems or threats of any kind, ready to turn on the stress response.

—10 Mindful Minutes

Sometimes fear can prevent us from taking any sort of action whatsoever. We feel incapacitated (that old amygdala takes over and skips past "fight" and "flight" to "freeze") because we're too overwhelmed.

For what is commonly called a "walking meditation," make sure that you have about ten minutes of uninterrupted time. No one should disturb you! Find a place where you can walk quietly: your backyard, around your living room—any space where you can just walk undistracted. As you walk, try to just focus on your breath. Just as with mindfulness breathing, the thoughts will come, but rather than trying to force them away, focus your attention on your steps, as each foot touches the ground and then you move ahead. Your only job is to pay attention to walking—almost as if you are walking for the first time.

the walking labyrinth

Throughout the world many people have created labyrinths designed specifically for walking meditations. They serve as a means for individuals to create a personal pilgrimage of sorts. Participants focus on movement along a particular path as they make their way toward the center, then return to the perimeter reflecting on what they have experienced, expressing gratitude for the journey and the insights they've received. Use a pen or pencil and enter the labyrinth. Keep the pencil moving and as you do this, try to keep your attention on what you're doing. Let any thoughts that arise pass by. Notice how you feel after doing this. (You may wish to photocopy this simple labyrinth and repeat the exercise whenever you feel the need.)

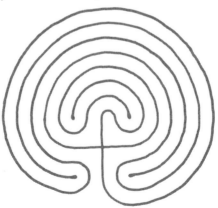

a letter to myself

You must approach your fears with as much truth
and courage as you can.

—A Lotus Grows in the Mud

There was a time in my life when I felt very reclusive. Fear kept me from fully participating in life. Yet I worked through what I was feeling and moved forward. We all have courage inside of us.

Write a letter to yourself about something that is making you fearful or holding you back. But write as though you are comforting a friend, a loved one, or a child about his or her fears. Our inner thoughts are sometimes our greatest ally. You'll be surprised at how empathetic you will feel—toward yourself and others—at the end of the letter.

discovering

empathy

*Practicing empathy is being tuned in and in tune to
the inner worlds of others and making an emotional
connection to that.*

—*10 Mindful Minutes*

I think we all have empathy. We may not have enough courage to display it.

—Maya Angelou

Have you ever heard the phrase "walk a mile in my shoes"? Or perhaps you've heard it sung by Elvis Presley! The expression nicely sums up empathy. Essentially, empathy means understanding how another person is feeling. You're connected to that person because you're both experiencing what emotion is being felt. You may be watching someone cry and feeling that sadness yourself. You might even cry. Or you may be watching the news and feeling the outrage that someone on television is displaying. It really is about being tuned in to another person's inner world as the quote above suggests. Try this empathy meditation below and deepen your connection to others.

1. Sit comfortably either in a chair or on a cushion. Make sure you're sitting nice and tall.

2. Place your palms faceup on top of your thighs.

3. Close your eyes and take a few deep inhales and exhales, settling into your body.

4. Observe the thoughts that arise, and let them drift off. Keep your attention on your breath.

5. When you feel ready, bring to mind the object of your empathy. This might be a person you know or a situation in your town, city, state, country, or elsewhere in the world. It might be an event going on in your own life. It can even be someone you don't know very well, such as your mail carrier, bank teller, or neighbor.

6. Say the following: "I wish [this person or this situation] to be free from suffering." Repeat silently while visualizing the person or situation for as long as it's comfortable.

really seeing someone

[Empathy] creates a greater capacity for tolerance, which diminishes the differences between us. We think beyond our own wants and needs and become curious about other people's.

—10 Mindful Minutes

Have you ever met someone for the first time and didn't really like them? Then as you found out more about them, and who they really are, you changed your mind and came to like them—or even love them? So often we pass judgments on people we don't even know. For the next thirty days, find one person a day and really look at him or her. It might be a stranger; it might be someone you know well or even someone with whom you have conflict. As you look at each person, imagine him or her as an innocent child. Remember, we were all once babes in arms. Then visualize this person being happy and carefree. Continue thinking about this person for a few minutes, really being present and seeing this person as another human being that you are connected to.

I suggest thirty days, which might seem a long time to you. However, research shows that it takes *at least* twenty-one days for something to become a habit. Certainly it takes time to change pathways in the brain. As well, I think doing this for another nine days could only be more beneficial to you! If you miss a day, don't worry; just pick up where you left off.

Take this opportunity to record your reflections on this exercise. You could focus on one or more individual encounters or on how *you* felt at the end of each week.

....

....

....

....

....

....

....

....

....

....

....

....

....

Empathy is a tool for building people into groups, for allowing us to function as more than self-obsessed individuals.

—Neil Gaiman

changing perspective

*Instead of being stuck in the drama of a situation,
we imagine being on the balcony in a movie theater watching
it like a film. From that distance, we can see the whole
picture and then find better solutions.*

—10 Mindful Minutes

To change your perspective about a situation, you sometimes need to take a fresh approach or look at it with a new pair of eyes. Think of a recent conflict you had with someone. Write about this conflict from *their* perspective. To really get into the other person's head, use the first person, "I" point of view. Then ask yourself, "What did I learn from this?"

What I learned from this exercise:

honoring connections

Every day, life presents us with opportunities to be compassionate, feel someone else's sadness or pain, and see things from another person's point of view.

—10 Mindful Minutes

"Let's get together soon!" "I'll call you." "I'll get right on that." "Let's grab a bite." How many of us have said these words to someone without the intention of ever following through? Or maybe we really do intend to spend time with that person but life gets in the way. It seems today we're all guilty of overcommitting. We've got families, work, kids, playdates, birthday parties . . . and the list goes on. But the question remains, how can we honor our connection to others without sacrificing our own needs? In the space provided below, first write out ways you can honor your own connections with others. I call this "Receiving Connections." Then write out some ideas on how you can honestly share whatever little time you have with others. I call this "Sharing Connections." I've put some examples down to help start the list.

RECEIVING CONNECTIONS

1. Allow time to have an uninterrupted conversation with a dear friend.

2. Listen to a compliment that someone pays you without deflecting it.

3. Pick up the phone instead of letting it go to voice mail.

4. ....

5. ....

6. ....

SHARING CONNECTIONS

1. Think of one small way to surprise a spouse, friend, or relative.

2. Suggest something fun to do with someone you enjoy spending time with.

3. Offer to do a favor for someone without any reciprocation involved.

4. ....

5. ....

6. ....

common humanity

Caring and empathy are necessary to build a healthy society.
—*10 Mindful Minutes*

Take a moment and think about the various people *closest to you* in your life: your spouse, your children, your relatives, your friends, and so on. Choose five important people. Then think about all the things you have in common with each person. Write down at least one thing or trait you share with that person.

1. ....

2. ....

3. ....

4. ....

5. ....

Now think of five people who you *don't know very well*. This might include your children's teacher, your spouse's boss, your boss, people you come in daily contact with but don't really socialize with. See if you can list two things you might have in common with these people. If you know nothing about a given person, take the time to find out a little more about him or her.

1. ....

2. ....

3. ....

4. ....

5. ....

The purpose of this journal entry is to try to see the common humanity that connects us all. Our social relationship circle tends to include those who share similar values, traits, and principles. That's wonderful; however, feeling more connected and empathetic toward those who we don't know very well or who appear to be "different" can be extremely liberating. Notice how you feel toward these five people after doing this entry. Has anything changed? Do you see the person differently? Record your feelings here.

....

....

becoming

compassionate

If we are to strive as human beings to gain more wisdom, more kindness, and more compassion, we must have the intention to grow as a lotus and open each petal one by one.

—The Nechung Oracle,
in *A Lotus Grows in the Mud*

Compassion is sometimes the fatal capacity for feeling what it is like to live inside somebody else's skin. It is the knowledge that there can never really be any peace and joy for me until there is peace and joy finally for you, too.

—Frederick Buechner

"Compassion" is a word often used to express the same *feeling* as empathy, yet the full expression of empathy is found in your desire to take action. In other words, you feel empathy *and* you want to do something to help others alleviate their pain—through acts of altruism.

This mindfulness moment will help to fulfill the intention of compassion within you—and set you on the path to action.

1. Sit comfortably either in a chair or on a cushion. Make sure you're sitting nice and tall.

2. Place your palms faceup on top of your thighs as a symbol of receiving.

3. Close your eyes and take a deep inhale; and as you exhale,

imagine your thoughts as clouds drifting across your mind. Try not to judge yourself or self-criticize or get caught up in your unresolved problems of the day.

4. Focus on your breath, at first being conscious of only your inhales and exhales. After a few breaths, when you feel calm yet energized, direct your thoughts toward a person or situation that is in need of your compassion.

5. Here are a few suggested phrases to start saying to yourself. Fill in the blanks with yourself or other people. You can create your own or use these.

"I hope .... receives everything he or she wants."

"I hope .... finds peace and happiness."

"I wish all the best for ...."

"May everyone find serenity and comfort."

self-compassion

By knowing and trusting in our goodness, we can free
ourselves to share that goodness with others. Then we create
a ripple effect emanating from our good deeds, spreading
even more empathy and joy.

—*10 Mindful Minutes*

I truly believe that one of the best ways to feel empathy and exercise
compassion is first to "put yourself in someone else's shoes" and then
to take action. This might be in the form of volunteering your time
for a worthwhile cause, sharing your knowledge with a student who's
struggling, helping a friend in need, or simply giving whatever you
can afford. However, some people, especially women, are such care-
takers and such doers that they forget to take care of themselves.

Just like the in-flight instructions to put on your own oxygen mask
before assisting others, we need to develop compassion for ourselves
before we can be truly caring to others.

Now is the time to celebrate yourself. Write some outrageous,
beautiful sentences that are in praise of you! For example: "I am the

most beautiful woman in the world." "I love the cellulite on my legs."
"What I'm doing right now is enough!"

Don't censor yourself, and forget the inner voice telling you differently.

pay it forward

*Resilience, self-understanding, and compassion are
essential skills that can be learned. In fact, learning and teaching
these skills may be what is necessary for us to shift the course
of human evolution in a more positive direction.*

—Daniel J. Siegel, MD, from the foreword to *10 Mindful Minutes*

Just thinking about compassion or a kind act can release dopamine, the hormone that is associated with positive emotions. You might even feel the sensation of warmth come over your body as you focus on putting someone else's needs before your own. Think about this quote: "If you want others to be happy, practice compassion. If you want to be happy, practice compassion."

Notice when someone shows you compassion. Perhaps someone allows you in a lane as you're driving, someone holds the door for you, or someone does a favor for you. Then you "pay it forward" by doing the same act or another act of compassion for someone else. Let's all put some positive energy and compassionate acts into our world!

Our human compassion binds us the one to the other—not in pity or patronizingly, but as human beings who have learnt how to turn our common suffering into hope for the future.

—Nelson Mandela

finding purpose

I've been dancing since I was three. I can honestly say that the highest points in my life, and when I've felt most joyful and integrated with everything around me, have been when I was moving my body to music. The method I learned required that we not only had to perform a pirouette, for instance, but also had to break down the movements to describe how each part of the body was connected to the next. It worked beautifully in integrating the two hemispheres of my brain and connecting my body and mind. On one night in particular, I was performing in West Side Story *in a theater in Baltimore. Time stood still. I felt I was dancing with the air, with the molecules of the unseen. I felt completely joyful, peaceful, purposeful, and exalted.*

—*10 Mindful Minutes*

How did compassion show up in your childhood? Were your parents compassionate? Did they show compassion toward you or others? Maybe you came from a family that, for whatever reason, was unable to show compassion. Developing a compassionate mind does not require that our parents pass this on to us. We can learn this at any stage of life. In her book *Lovingkindness: The Revolutionary Art of*

Happiness, Buddhist author and teacher Sharon Salzberg writes, "The first step in developing true compassion is being able to recognize, to open to, and to acknowledge that pain and sorrow exist." This does not mean that we need to dwell in others' suffering but simply acknowledge it.

One of the simplest ways to develop compassion is to find purpose in something where others will benefit—a compassionate act of service. Below, consider what purpose you can bring into your own life and something that will help others. For example, you might find purpose in volunteering for a few hours in your child's classroom.

the garden of compassion

One truth we can be sure of: praying for someone's well-being while they are still on this earth, by reaching out and trying to help them in any way we can, by developing more compassion in our hearts and in our lives and in our spirits, will help make a better world.

—*A Lotus Grows in the Mud*

Rumi was a thirteenth-century Persian theologian and poet whose works are passionate and profound. Read the quote from his work below and then write freely about what this quote means to you. What feelings arise? How is this connected to compassion for you? How do you keep your heart open?

Grief can be the garden of compassion. If you keep your heart open through everything, your pain can become your greatest ally in your life's search for love and wisdom.

nurturing words

Each of us goes through transitions and transformations.
The important thing is that we acknowledge them and
learn from them.

—A Lotus Grows in the Mud

Every major religion or spiritual practice contains the idea that one should not harm others. And certainly, a compassionate person tries to live up to this principle. Of course, we're all human and we make mistakes. Hopefully we learn from them. Harming others can also include how we talk to others and gossip about others. His Holiness the Dalai Lama XIV said, "If you can, help others; if you cannot do that, at least do not harm them."

In the space provided below, be honest about how you talk about others. Are your words truthful and kind? Would you say the exact same thing directly to that person? Let's nurture our words and feed the goodness that lies in us all.

How I speak about my spouse to others:

....

....

....

....

....

How I speak about my friends to others:

....

....

....

....

....

How I speak about people I don't know very well:

....

....

....

....

....

How I speak about my parents:

....
....
....
....
....

How I speak about my relatives:

....
....
....
....
....

If there are other people not listed above, include them below:

....
....
....
....
....

tending to
kindness

In an ideal world, we should all be drawn to acts of kindness whether or not we think it is good for us.

—*10 Mindful Minutes*

*A tree is known by its fruit; a man by
his deeds. A good deed is never lost; he who sows
courtesy reaps friendship, and he who
plants kindness gathers love.*

—Saint Basil

A discussion about kindness naturally follows the empathy and compassion sections because kindness comes from thinking about others. During this mindful breathing time, create the intention of seeing, feeling, and experiencing kindness in all areas of your life.

1. Sit comfortably either in a chair or on a cushion. Make sure you're sitting nice and tall.

2. Place your palms facedown on top of your thighs. This will help ground you.

3. Close your eyes and take a deep inhale; and as you exhale, observe your thoughts floating through your mind.

4. Focus on your breath, your inhales and exhales.

5. When you feel ready, bring to mind a kind act that someone has done for you. Thank that person as you recall this event.

6. Bring to mind a kind act you have done for someone. Recall how good you felt at that moment.

7. Keep going, switching between thinking about a kind gesture someone has done for you and one that you have done for someone.

8. Just be aware of how you feel and cherish the potential for kindness within you—and others.

acts of kindness

According to psychologist Sonja Lyubomirsky, doing just five small acts of kindness a week can boost our moods, particularly if we do a variety of them all in one day.

—10 Mindful Minutes

Sometimes it is hard to feel kindness when we're having a bad day, week, or even month! The good news is that you can change how you feel simply by doing something you might not want to do. Research has shown that even the act of smiling triggers a psychological response and we feel happier. Do you notice that when someone smiles at you, you instinctively smile back?

No matter how you're feeling, set an intention of doing five small random acts of kindness during the week. It may be as simple as smiling at someone. It may be doing a favor for a friend. Whatever it is, helping others will make you feel good.

At the end of the week come back to this page to record and reflect upon these random acts of kindness, whether you gave them anonymously (which is, some say, the best) or not. And, perhaps equally important, what acts of kindness did you experience from others that might have been prompted by your initiative?

kindness all around

Accepting that we have the capacity to be kind allows us to go out into the world as adults with a sense of optimism and value.

—*10 Mindful Minutes*

How have you seen kindness today? List all the kind acts you saw and include your own. Do this for seven days and notice how you start seeing more and more kindness around you. Kindness begets kindness!

DAY 1

....

....

....

....

....

DAY 2

DAY 3

DAY 4

DAY 5

....

....

....

....

....

DAY 6

....

....

....

....

....

DAY 7

....

....

....

....

....

who do you admire?

When will we learn that it doesn't matter which tribe we belong to? When will we understand that we all belong to the greatest tribe there is: the human race?

—A Lotus Grows in the Mud

Think about someone you admire because of their kindness—a friend, colleague, or famous person. How have they demonstrated kindness? What do you think motivates them when so many others may not be so obviously kind? Write about this person, perhaps in the form of a letter expressing your admiration.

receiving

*Every relationship is a gift. . . . What great gifts I have
been given by each of the people I have encountered on my
journey through life. How they have helped shape me into
the person I have become and still hope to be.*

—A Lotus Grows in the Mud

Human beings are social creatures. Even if you consider yourself an
introvert, we do depend upon others in some way. And part of the
beauty of life includes encountering people who help us out along
the way. Sometimes their kind acts are small, yet they may have the
greatest impact upon us. People may also show extraordinary kindness toward us, bringing us to tears.

What is the kindest gesture or act that someone has ever done for
you? Think about this for a few minutes. Recall your life and then
write about how this kindness affected you. How did it alter your
life? Your perspective? How does it make you feel now to think about
it? Receive the feelings that arise and be open to experiencing that
gratitude you feel.

talk about it

I don't believe there is such a thing as a perfect parent.
I know that I'm still on my own journey of development and
growth as a human being, even though my children are now
adults. All we can hope is that our children experience
more positive than negative effects from our parenting
and become the healthy pilots of their own lives.

—*10 Mindful Minutes*

Being an example for our children is one of the most important roles of our lives as parents. And while being a role model for kindness is vital, you still need to talk with your children about kindness as a simple way to water the seed of kindness that you've planted by your example. Have daily dinner conversations about kindness. Ask your children how they were kind that day. Share with them how you were kind. Let this be a continual ongoing conversation that allows your children to blossom.

journaling your way to a more mindful life

As I mentioned in the introduction, I believe that what we think is what we create. Writing down our thoughts, inner feelings, and reflections can be a powerful transformative tool. It is possible to channel all that we think into something more aligned with the inner light that exists in us all. Sometimes we don't even realize how our inner critic affects all that we manifest. By using these meditations and journal prompts, you will discover that no matter what age you are, it is always possible to realize your fullest potential.

Part of being mindful and taking time to write down your thoughts means reflecting upon what you discover about yourself. This might be scary at times, but as the Buddha said, "Three things cannot be long hidden: the sun, the moon, and the truth" (paraphrased). Embrace all that you are, including the parts that you don't like. I think one of the greatest gifts that comes from writing is being able to see a different perspective. It's like some sort of magic happens when we take pen to paper. We are cultivating a power of awareness.

When we take the time to nurture ourselves and fearlessly embark on a journey to know ourselves better, the universe never, ever disappoints. What you will get back is virtually impossible to put into words. Your world will open up and you will see things differently. Your attitude and outlook will change because you have retrained your brain to think differently. I know because it's worked for me!

If you truly take a few minutes to do these mindful practices, you will start to notice how much more calm you feel on a daily basis. You might pause and take a breath when you feel agitated, then be able to separate yourself from your negative thoughts, creating more awareness to react differently. By sitting quietly, following the meditation exercises, you are creating space *between* your thoughts. Stress leads to more illness. By living a more mindful life, you will see your health improve. Be a witness to how your own mindful practice affects those around you. If you're calmer, those around you will most likely become calmer, too.

Finally, the journal pages at the end of this book are included for you to keep journaling about whatever you wish. Use it daily, a few times a week, or however often doing so fits your life.

Take ownership of your life, your future, and your own personal growth. Use this place where you write your thoughts down as *your* place. It's personal, it's private, and it's the beginning of a journey to create a happier, healthier, more mindful life. Have fun!

Date: ....

Today I ....

....

....

....

....

....

....

....

....

....

....

....

....

....

....

....

....

....

....

....

....

....

Date: ....

Today I ....

Date:

Today I

Date: ....

Today I ....

....

....

....

....

....

....

....

....

....

....

....

....

....

....

....

....

....

....

....

....

....

Date: ....

Today I ....

....

....

....

....

....

....

....

....

....

....

....

....

....

....

....

....

....

....

Date:..

Today I ....

....

....

....

....

....

....

....

....

....

....

....

....

....

....

....

....

....

....

....

....

Date:

Today I

Date: ....

Today I ....

....

....

....

....

....

....

....

....

....

....

....

....

....

....

....

....

....

....

....

....

Date:

Today I

Date: ....

Today I ....

....

....

....

....

....

....

....

....

....

....

....

....

....

....

....

....

....

....

....

Date: ....

Today I ....

....

....

....

....

....

....

....

....

....

....

....

....

....

....

....

....

....

....

Date: ....

Today I ....

Date: ....

Today I ....

....

....

....

....

....

....

....

....

....

....

....

....

....

....

....

....

....

....

....

....

....

Date: ....

Today I ....

....

....

....

....

....

....

....

....

....

....

....

....

....

....

....

....

....

....

Date: ....

Today I ....

....

....

....

....

....

....

....

....

....

....

....

....

....

....

....

....

....

....

....

Date:

Today I

Date: ....

Today I ....

....

....

....

....

....

....

....

....

....

....

....

....

....

....

....

....

....

....

....

....

Date: ....

Today I ....

....

....

....

....

....

....

....

....

....

....

....

....

....

....

....

....

....

....

....

Date: ....

Today I ....

....

....

....

....

....

....

....

....

....

....

....

....

....

....

....

....

....

....

Date:

Today I

Date:

Today I

Date: ....

Today I ....

....

....

....

....

....

....

....

....

....

....

....

....

....

....

....

....

....

....

....

Date: ....

Today I ....
....
....
....
....
....
....
....
....
....
....
....
....
....
....
....
....
....
....

Date: ....

Today I ....
....
....
....
....
....
....
....
....
....
....
....
....
....
....
....
....
....
....
....
....
....

Date:

Today I

Date: ....

Today I ....

....

....

....

....

....

....

....

....

....

....

....

....

....

....

....

....

....

....

....

....

Date: ....

Today I ....

....

....

....

....

....

....

....

....

....

....

....

....

....

....

....

....

....

....

....

....

Date:

Today I

Date: ....

Today I ....

....

....

....

....

....

....

....

....

....

....

....

....

....

....

....

....

....

....

....

....

....

....

Date: ....

Today I ....

....

....

....

....

....

....

....

....

....

....

....

....

....

....

....

....

....

....

....

Date: ....

Today I ....

....

....

....

....

....

....

....

....

....

....

....

....

....

....

....

....

....

....

....

Date: ....

Today I ....

....

....

....

....

....

....

....

....

....

....

....

....

....

....

....

....

....

....

....

....

Date: ....

Today I ....

....

....

....

....

....

....

....

....

....

....

....

....

....

....

....

....

....

....

....

Date: ....

Today I ....

....

....

....

....

....

....

....

....

....

....

....

....

....

....

....

....

....

....

....

Date: ....

Today I ....

....

....

....

....

....

....

....

....

....

....

....

....

....

....

....

....

....

....

....

Date: ....

Today I ....

....

....

....

....

....

....

....

....

....

....

....

....

....

....

....

....

....

Date: ....

Today I ....

....

....

....

....

....

....

....

....

....

....

....

....

....

....

....

....

....

....

Date: ....

Today I ....

....

....

....

....

....

....

....

....

....

....

....

....

....

....

....

....

....

Date: ....

Today I ....

....

....

....

....

....

....

....

....

....

....

....

....

....

....

....

....

....

....

Date: ....

Today I ....

Date: ....

Today I ....

....

....

....

....

....

....

....

....

....

....

....

....

....

....

....

....

....

....

Date: ....

Today I ....

....

....

....

....

....

....

....

....

....

....

....

....

....

....

....

....

....

....

....

Date: ....

Today I ....

....

....

....

....

....

....

....

....

....

....

....

....

....

....

....

....

....

....

....

Date: ....

Today I ....

....

....

....

....

....

....

....

....

....

....

....

....

....

....

....

....

....

....

....

Date: ....

Today I ....

....

....

....

....

....

....

....

....

....

....

....

....

....

....

....

....

....

....

Date:

Today I

Date: ....

Today I ....

....

....

....

....

....

....

....

....

....

....

....

....

....

....

....

....

....

....

....

....

....

Date: ....

Today I ....

....

....

....

....

....

....

....

....

....

....

....

....

....

....

....

....

....

....

....

Date: ....

Today I ....

....

....

....

....

....

....

....

....

....

....

....

....

....

....

....

....

....

....

Date: ....

Today I ....

....

....

....

....

....

....

....

....

....

....

....

....

....

....

....

....

....

....

....

Date:

Today I

Date: ....

Today I ....

....

....

....

....

....

....

....

....

....

....

....

....

....

....

....

....

....

....

....

Date:

Today I

Date:

Today I

Date: ....

Today I ....

....

....

....

....

....

....

....

....

....

....

....

....

....

....

....

....

....

....

....

Date: ....

Today I ....

....

....

....

....

....

....

....

....

....

....

....

....

....

....

....

....

....

....

....

....

....

Date: ....

Today I ....

....

....

....

....

....

....

....

....

....

....

....

....

....

....

....

....

....

....

....

....

Date:...

Today I ....

....

....

....

....

....

....

....

....

....

....

....

....

....

....

....

....

....

....

....

....

Date: ....

Today I ....

....

....

....

....

....

....

....

....

....

....

....

....

....

....

....

....

....

....

....

....

Date: ....

Today I ....

Date: ....

Today I ....

....

....

....

....

....

....

....

....

....

....

....

....

....

....

....

....

....

....

Date: ....

Today I ....

....

....

....

....

....

....

....

....

....

....

....

....

....

....

....

....

....

....

....

....

Date: ....

Today I ....

....

....

....

....

....

....

....

....

....

....

....

....

....

....

....

....

....

....

....

....

....

Date: ....

Today I ....

....

....

....

....

....

....

....

....

....

....

....

....

....

....

....

....

....

....

Date: ....

Today I ....

....

....

....

....

....

....

....

....

....

....

....

....

....

....

....

....

....

....

....

....

....

Date: ....

Today I ....

....

....

....

....

....

....

....

....

....

....

....

....

....

....

....

....

....

....

....

Date: ....

Today I ....

....

....

....

....

....

....

....

....

....

....

....

....

....

....

....

....

....

....

....

Date: ....

Today I ....

....

....

....

....

....

....

....

....

....

....

....

....

....

....

....

....

....

....

....

about the author

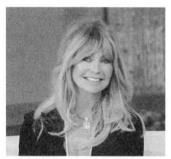

Goldie Hawn is the founder of the Hawn Foundation as well as an international children's advocate and enthusiastic campaigner for the mindful celebration of life. An Academy Award–winning actress, producer, and director, she is also a mother and grandmother. Her bestselling memoir, *A Lotus Grows in the Mud*, was published in 2005. Her second book, *10 Mindful Minutes*, published in 2011, was also a *New York Times* and international bestseller.

TheHawnFoundation.org
Twitter: @goldiehawn
Facebook: Goldie Hawn

1 800
900 - 4248